The Palette of Breath

Facts About Breathing

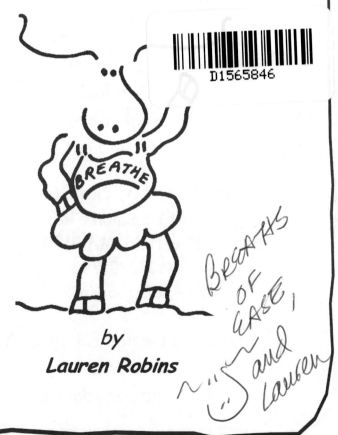

by
Lauren Robins

BREATHS OF EASE,
~ :) and Lauren

ISBN 1-884820-77-8
3rd Printing, Revised Edition
Printed in the United States of America

Library of Congress Control Number:
2004092819

The Palette of Breath is not intended as medical advice. It is written solely for informational and educational purposes. Please consult a health professional should the need for one be indicated.

Published by Safe Goods
561 Shunpike Rd.
Sheffield, MA 01257
413-229-7935
www.safegoodspub.com

Graphic Design & Layout by
Joe Stack
www.embeddedart.com

This book is dedicated
to all my relations
and the breath of kindness
within us all.

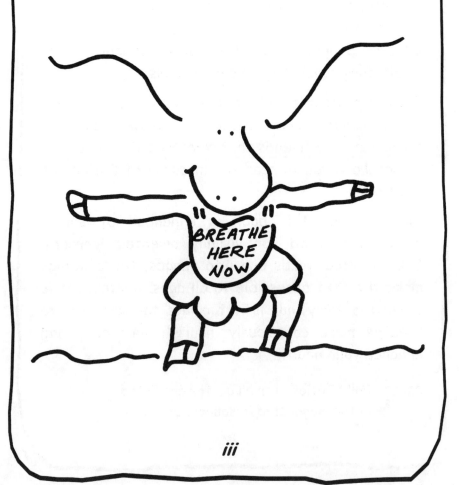

Foreword

Breathing Life into This Book

As a massage therapist and movement educator for twenty years, I have been keeping a pulse on the benefits of conscious breathing. During this time, I have seen a profound increase in the number of books, research articles, interviews and web sites addressing the magnificent advantages of breathing awareness. We can now point to data by doctors, professional caregivers, therapists, educators, fitness experts, athletes, yoga teachers and meditators supporting this awareness.

I am in gratitude and am held in awe upon hearing the amazing stories from my clients, teachers, caregivers and friends that reinforce this research. I encourage you to read the message at the end of the text.

The text of this book is enhanced by simple drawings created for visually oriented learners. Going beyond words and into images, the drawings make the text accessible to all ages. Certainly it is never too early, nor is it too late to learn how to breathe more consciously, nourish your body and enhance your health.

Note: Full citations for all quotes are listed in the Suggested Resources section.

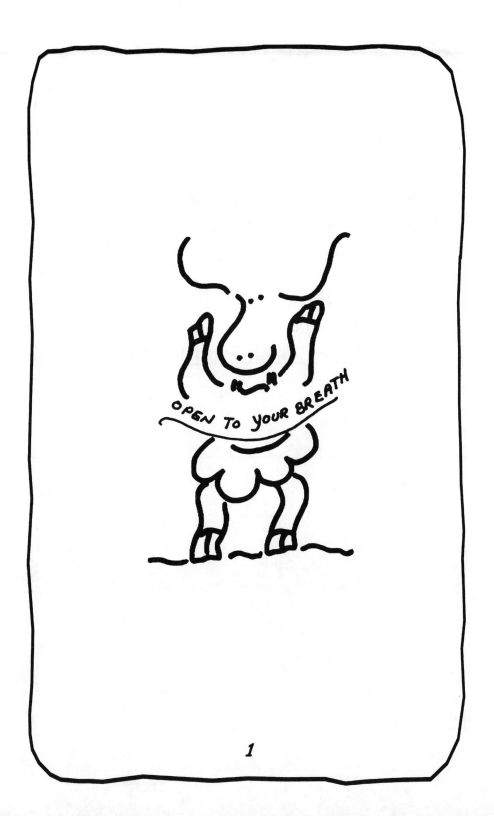

"Often we don't know we're tensing our abdomens, and the muscular tension becomes chronic."

~*Alice Domar, PhD. &*
  Henry Dreher
  <u>Healing Mind, Healthy Woman</u>

Hello,

I invite you to enjoy the breaths you take while learning from this book.

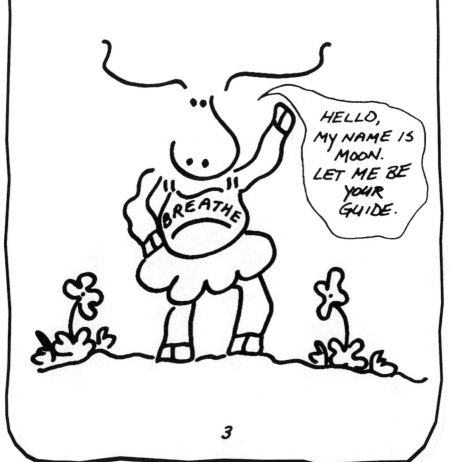

"Draw a picture of yourself, your heart, your lungs and your diaphragm. Enhance it with color and pleasing words or symbols."

~MOON

This book is entitled <u>The Palette of Breath</u> because just as a palette holds the colors selected by the artist for the work, your breath is the palette holding the physical, mental, emotional, and spiritual colors you select to create yourself. How you color your breath is who you are in the world. The actions and the intention behind your breath determine your palette of health.

I invite you to color and doodle in this book and use it as a journal of breath.

OPEN TO YOUR BREATH

5

"Your breath is in your blood."

~MOON

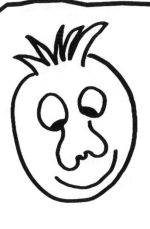 There it is right under your nose, your necessary number one food - your breath.

Awareness of its nourishment will enhance the way that you creatively support and nurture yourself.

It's worked well for me.

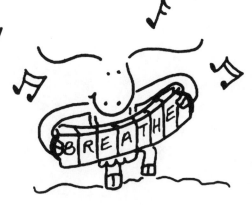

"We can learn to use the breath as a Geiger Counter to sense, locate, and define our experience."

~Donna Farhi
   The Breathing Book

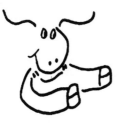

Here are some words to help you read this book

■ ‥ ■ ‥ ■ ‥ ■ ‥ ■

Inhale
&
Exhale

> *To breathe - comes from an Old English word meaning healthy and holy.*

Diaphragm — *Muscular membrane completely separating upper and lower parts of the body. Its movement empties and fills the lungs, expanding the ribs and the belly button.*

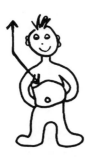

♥ = *Heart*
O_2 = *Oxygen (Inhaled)*
CO_2 = *Carbon Dioxide (Exhaled)*

9

"It is mostly pointless to breathe into the high chest because there is very little lung volume there."

~Michael Grant White
The Breathing Coach
The Optimal Breathing School,
Executive Director

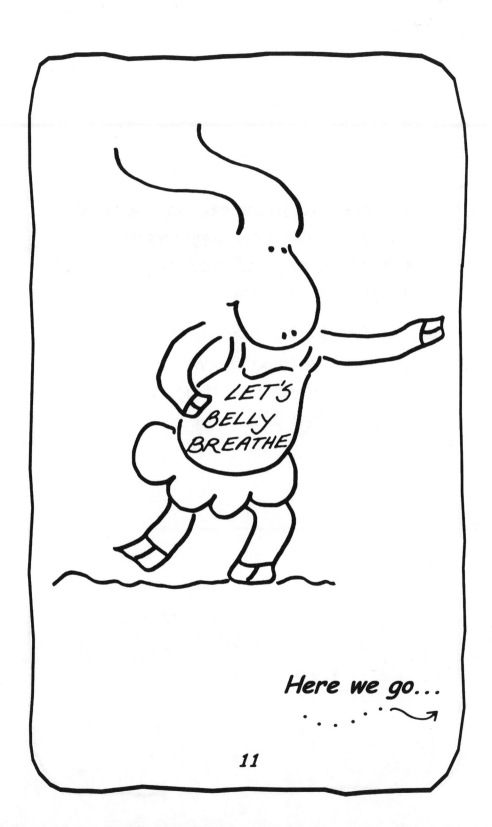

"For over 30 years exciting data has been collected that supports the importance of good breathing for peak health and longevity."

~Michael Grant White
The Breathing Coach
The Optimal Breathing School,
Executive Director

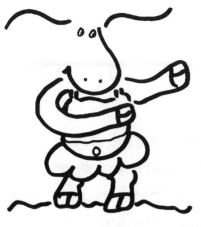

This way to easy belly breathing...

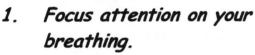

1. Focus attention on your breathing.

2. Listen to your breathing for a few moments.

3. Without any strain, easily and consciously exhale (through your nose if possible). Bring your belly back toward your spine.

4. Without any strain, easily and consciously inhale (through your nose if possible). Inhale into all parts of your diaphragm. A round belly is good.

5. Enjoy a gentle pause, a stillness, in between the exhale and the inhale.

13

"There is no substitute for the creative inspiration, knowledge and stability that comes from knowing how to contact your inner silence."

~Deepak Chopra, MD.
   <u>Ageless Body Timeless Mind</u>

As you continue, why not become friends with your breath? Remember, it's your number one life source.

Then to enhance your life source, flood your breath with peace... or song... or whatever you're needing right now.

SEE IF YOU CAN DO THIS BREATHING SEVERAL TIMES A DAY.

15

"Life is the breath.
He who half breathes, half lives."

~Ancient Eastern proverb

Easy belly breathing is healthy because...
each breath refreshes your body.

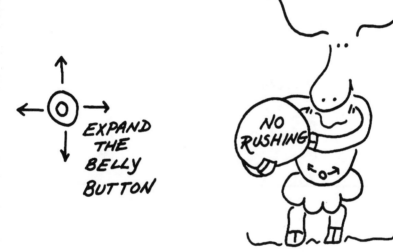

EXPAND
THE
BELLY
BUTTON

NO RUSHING

Many of us have the capacity to inhale up to 4 quarts of air; most of us breathe in only 2 pints.

"Laughter causes a decrease in blood pressure and an increase in growth hormones."

~Lee Berk, DrPH
The Science of Laughter (CD-ROM)

Easy belly breathing is healthy because...

it allows you to belly laugh.

Laughing brings more O_2 to the body, flooding it with healthy yummies.*

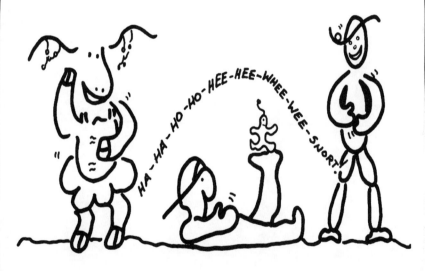

*Yummies = chemicals that make your immune system stronger. Tah-Dah!!

"The diaphragm is also known as the second heart."

~Mabel Todd
  The Thinking Body

Easy belly breathing is healthy because...

it massages your organs.

One of the organs massaged with each breath is the ♥.

Did you know there are muscles connecting the ♥* to the diaphragm?

* The muscle sac around the ♥ is connected to every inhale and exhale.

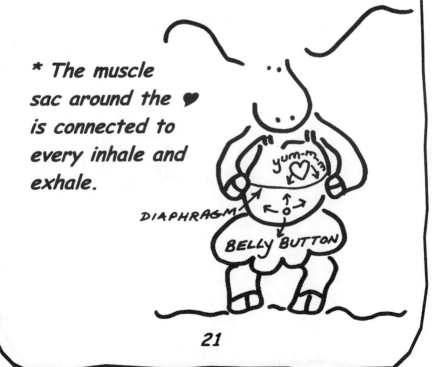

DIAPHRAGM

yum-mm

BELLY BUTTON

"For high blood pressure, 'The Meninger Foundation, in Kansas, uses deep breathing...90 percent of the Foundation's high-blood-pressure patients shift their pressure to normal range' using this technique."

~James Loehr, EdD. &
Jeffrey Migdow, M.D.
Breath In Breath Out

Easy belly breathing is healthy because...

it can lower your blood pressure.

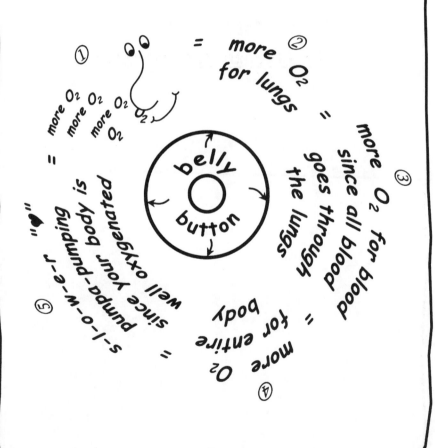

① more O_2 more O_2 more O_2 O_2

= more O_2 for lungs ②

= more O_2 for blood since all blood goes through the lungs ③

= more O_2 for entire body ④

= s-l-o-w-e-r "❤" pumpa-pumping is since your body is well oxygenated ⑤

belly button

"Breathing is the first place not the last place one should investigate when any disordered energy presents itself."

~Sheldon Saul Handler
   The Oxygen Breakthrough

Easy belly breathing is healthy because...

it also massages the vessels carrying blood, lymph and food.

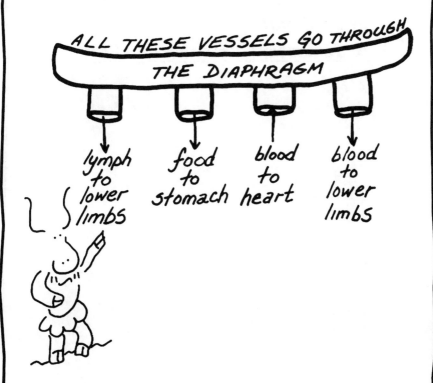

ALL THESE VESSELS GO THROUGH THE DIAPHRAGM

lymph to lower limbs

food to stomach

blood to heart

blood to lower limbs

Tension in the diaphragm can cause digestive problems.

"...the one element that all successful weight loss programs had in common... oxygen, pure and simple."

~Pam Grout
<u>Jumpstart Your Metabolism</u>

Easy belly breathing is healthy because...

it can assist you in controlling weight.

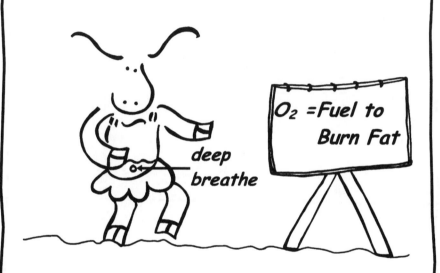

Billions of cells are burned daily. 70 percent of the body's wastes are processed through breathing.

"The breath acts as a steadfast and loyal servant of the body, endlessly offering its life-giving energy to the bloodstream."

~*Irene Ringawa*
   Darshan Magazine

*Easy belly breathing is
healthy because...*

*it gives you the space and time
to calm your mind.*

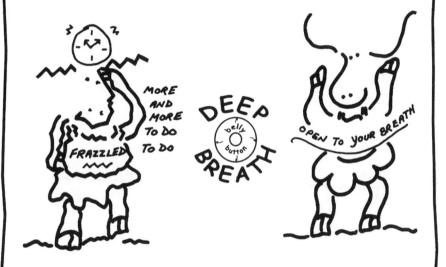

*An overstressed nervous system
steals oxygen from other parts
of your body.*

"A merry heart does good like medicine, but a heavy heart drieth the bone."

   ~Old Testament

*Easy belly breathing is
healthy because...*

*it allows you to be aware
of your emotions.*

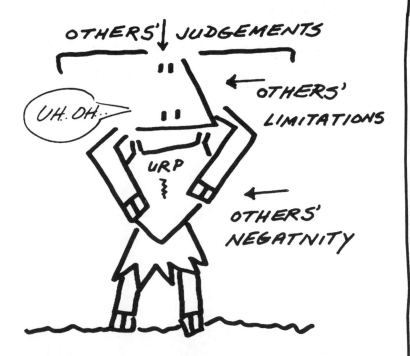

*Shallow breathing — resulting
from fear, anger, shame and
guilt — can deplete your body
of its nutrients.*

"There are about 75 trillion cells in your body and they are all breathing-or should be."

~Sheldon Saul Handler, MD., PhD.
The Oxygen Breakthrough

Easy belly breathing is
healthy because...

it sends O_2 to your muscles
and joints as you
stretch and play.

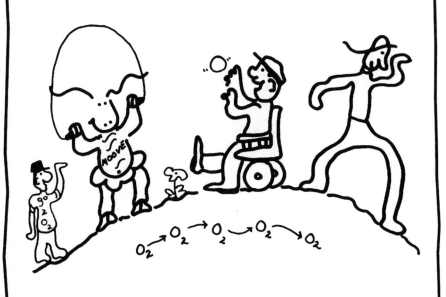

Sometimes aches and pains are
caused by shallow breathing.

".Breath control is the force that leads to the emotional control that leads to the winning feat...mental control will be heightened by this process."

~James Loehr, EdD. &
Jeffrey Migdow, MD
Take a Deep Breath

Easy belly breathing is
healthy because...

it helps increase athletic
performance.

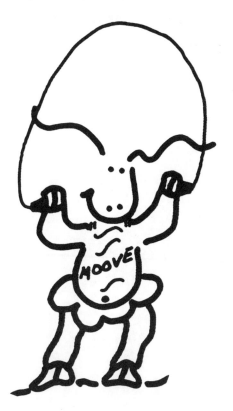

Endurance is enhanced and sports
injuries are lessened.

"The simplest and most important technique for protecting your health is breathing."

~Andrew Weil, MD
<u>Spontaneous Healing</u>

Easy belly breathing is healthy because...

it balances your acid-alkaline ratio.

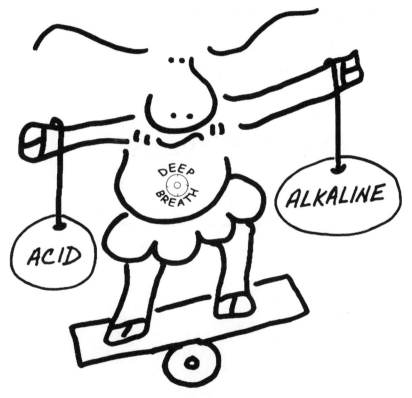

Shallow breathing creates more acid in your body. Viruses grow in an overly acidic environment.

"...breathing can help you develop to the utmost, enabling you to acquire a greater sense of power and balance and to sharpen both your mental and physical coordination."

~Nancy Zi
   The Art of Breathing

Easy belly breathing is healthy because...

it can calm your mind and give you time to listen to your interior healing voice.

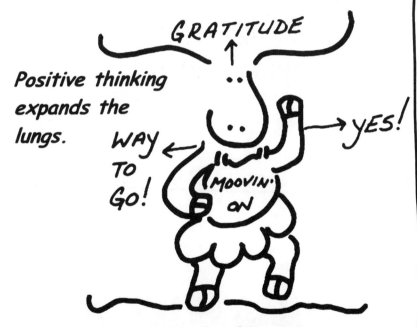

Your interior healing voice = your interior decorator

Deep easy exhalations invite deep easy inhalations.

"Meditation has been helping in treating irregular heart rhythms... lowering cholesterol levels... and reducing attacks of angina."

~Larry Dosey, MD.
Meaning and Medicine

Deep easy belly breathing is
healthy because...

it deepens meditation.

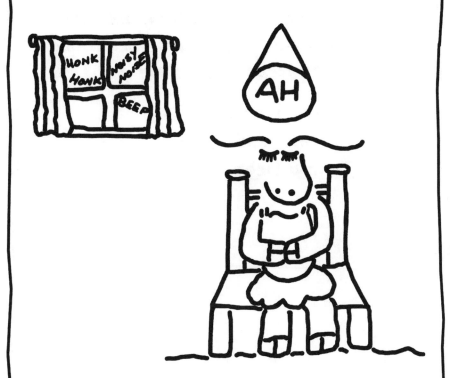

Meditation gives way to healing.

"The power of breath is awesome. Many accomplished singers, musicians, dancers and actors employ breathing techniques to perfect their art."

~James Loehr, EdD. & Jeffrey Migdow, MD
Take a Deep Breath

*Easy belly breathing is
healthy and entertaining because...*

it allows you to...

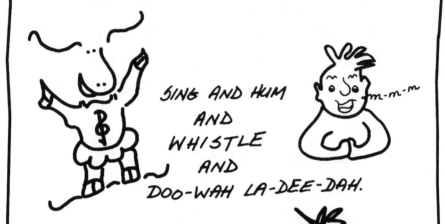

*This vibrates every
cell with your own music* · · ·
strengthening your immune system.

43

"We have only so much energy with which to run our lives, and using that energy to run our past (or future) more than our present causes us to run into energetic debt."

~Carolyn Myss, PhD
   <u>**Why People Don't Heal**</u>
   <u>**and How They Can**</u>

*Easy belly breathing is
healthy because...*

*it reminds you to be
present in each moment.*

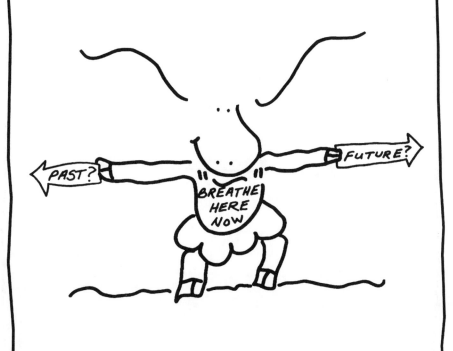

"Cover your ears and listen to your breathing. It will teach you many lessons."

~MOON

Four Questions to Consider About Your Breathing:

1. How did I entertain my breath today?

2. Did I breathe with more awareness today?

3. Did I bring a compassionate breath to someone else today?

4. When my breath whispered in my ear today, did I listen?

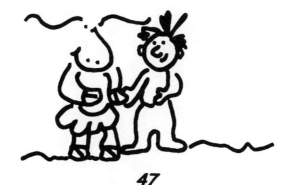

"As the universe breathes into you, let yourself feel the breath penetrating to every part of your body, even the tips of your fingers and toes."

~Andrew Weil, MD
Spontaneous Healing

And remember, easy belly breathing is healthy because...

through breathing you experience your connection with nature.

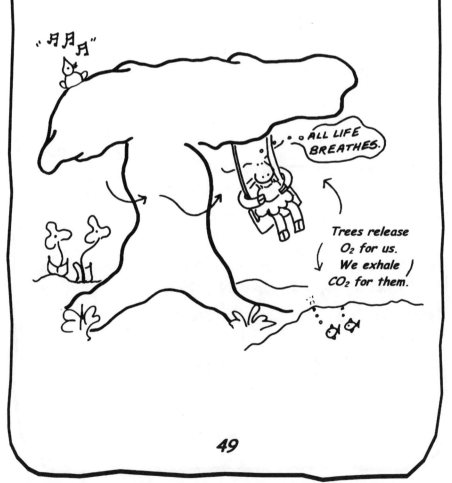

Suggested Resources
Books on Breathing

Berk, DrPH., Lee · *The Science of Laughter: An Introduction* ·
   CD ROM, An Interview on NPR circa 2000 ·
   www.drleeberk.com

Brody, Jane & Gray, Denise ·
   The New York Times' Guide to Alternative Health ·
   Times Books, New York, NY · 2001

Chopra, Deepak · *Ageless Body, Timeless Mind* ·
   Crown/Random House, New York, NY · 1993

Domar, PhD., Alice & Dreher, Henry · *Healing Mind,*
   Healthy Woman ·
   Holt, New York, NY · 1996

Dosey, MD, Larry · *Meaning and Medicine* ·
   Bantam/Dell, New York, NY · 1991

Farhi, Donna · *The Breathing Book* ·
   Simon & Schuster, New York, NY · 1997

Grout, Pam · *Jumpstart Your Metabolism* ·
   Scribner, Riverside, NJ · 1996

Handler, MD, PhD, Sheldon Saul · *The Oxygen Breakthrough* ·
   Pocket Books, Old Tappan, NJ · 1991

Hendricks, PhD., Gay · *Conscious Breathing* ·
   Bantam, New York, NY · 1995

Iyengar, B.K.S. · *Yoga, The Path to Holistic Health* ·
   Dorling Kindersley, London, England · 2001

Suggested Resources

(Continued...)

Loehr, EdD., James, & Migdow, MD, Jeffery ·
    Breathe In , Breathe Out ·
    Time/Life, Boston, MA · 1999

Loehr, EdD., James, & Migdow, MD, Jeffery ·
    Take a Deep Breath ·
    Villard Books, New York, NY · 1986

Myss, PhD., Carolyn ·
    Why People Don't Heal and How They Can ·
    Three Rivers Press, New York, NY · 1997

Ringawa, Irene · *Darshan, "It's All in the Breath"* ·
    South Fallsburg, NY · March, 1993

Swami Rama, Ballentine & Hymes ·
    The Science of Breathing ·
    Holt, New York, NY · 1996

Speads , Carola · *Breathing the ABC's* ·
    Harper, New York, NY · 1978

Todd, Mabel · *The Thinking Body* ·
    Princeton Book, Ewing, NJ, · 1972

Weil, Andrew · *Spontaneous Healing* ·
    Fawcett, Westminster, MD · 2000

White, Michael Grant · The Breathing Coach ·
    www.breathing.com

Zi, Nancy · *The Art of Breathing* ·
    Bantam, New York, NY · 1986

More Suggested Resources

Books on Creativity and the Body

Chia, Mantak • *Chi Self Massage* •
Healing Tao Books, Huntington, NY • 1986

Hahn, Thich Naht • *Present Moment, Wonderful
Moment* • Parallax Press, Berkley, CA • 1990

Halprin, Anna • *Dance as a Healing Art* •
Life Rhythm, Mendocino, CA • 2000

Mettler, Barbara • *Dance as an Element of Life* •
Mettler Studios, Inc., Tucson, AZ • 1983

Nachmanovitch, Stephen • *Free Play* •
Jeremy Tarcher, Inc.,
New York, NY • 1990

Northrup, Christine, M.D. •
Women's Bodies, Women's Wisdom •
Bantam, New York, NY • 1991

Pert, Candace • *Molecules of Emotion* •
Simon & Schuster,
New York, NY • 1999

Sarno, John, M.D. •
Healing Back Pain • Warner Books,
New York, NY • 1991

Web Sites

www.breathing.com (just search for "Breathing")

52

MOON is a whimsical cow who likes to help people. She can be heard saying, "If I don't see you in the future, I'll see you in the pasture".

Lauren Robins, M.S. in Special Education and Licensed Massage Therapist, has enjoyed and taught in the pastures of improvisational and post-modern dance, voice, massage therapy, yoga, and doodling. Presently, she is breathing in the Texas Hill Country and leading seminars on breath and mooovement. To get in touch with MOON or Lauren, contact us at lrobins2000@yahoo.com.

MESSAGE TO HEALTH CARE PROFESSIONALS, EDUCATORS AND CARE GIVERS

In our high paced society, with stress being one of the main reasons for disease, it is necessary that we turn our attention inward to our breath. Studies have shown that slow, mindful, deep breathing reduces stress thus calming the nervous system. Once the nervous system is calmed the health of the body, mind and spirit is elevated.

Healthcare professionals, educators and care givers have shared stories informing me of the benefits of reading and sharing this book. It has aided doctors in their interactions with patients. Deepak Chopra, M.D. writes in Ageless Body, Timeless Mind, "As a young intern on duty in the emergency room, I was taught to calm down agitated patients just by sitting next to them and asking them to breathe slowly, deeply, and regularly along with me. As we fell into a relaxed breathing rhythm, our bodies spontaneously followed suit, and their agitated emotions were stilled." Other doctors and dentists use the deep breathing technique before, during and after procedures.

Nurses have talked about the positive effects of deep breathing. They have found deep breathing useful when administering vaccinations, and, of course, in childbirth. School nurses see a rise in student visitations at test time when anxiety levels are high. After deep breathing with the students for only a few moments, most students return to the classroom reportedly feeling more in control and less jittery.

Elementary educators have been gathering with their classes at the beginning, middle and end of the school day creating a feeling of community as they breathe together. One fifth grade teacher shared with me that she has a "Breathing Corner" in the classroom. Children go there whenever they feel out of balance. To date, she has had no fights in her classroom and test results have improved. Other teachers have found positive results using the deep breathing technique before testing procedures or before public speaking assignments.

54

Care givers, be they family members or therapists, also comment that by reading and sharing this book, a bond has been created with those they are helping. Both parties have become more aware of the profound results of slow, deep belly breathing as a calming and free bit of medicine. Plus, learning more of the facts about breathing has accentuated the immediate and lasting results.

At my seminars or after having read <u>The Palette of Breath</u>, people of all ages and from all walks of life have repeatedly offered the following feedback.

"I am not aware of my breathing at all."

"I wish I knew this information years ago especially in dealing with my aging parents. No one's ever taught me this. And it's so important. It's helped with raising my children too."

"Oh, I never breathe...or I catch myself holding my breath a lot."

"I am slowly developing an awareness of my breathing. I'm beginning to realize how many times a day I can use this information."

"Your book has made me realize that when I breathe deeply, my posture improves."

"This book is refreshing because it's so easy to read. I love the drawings. I actually want to breathe deeper."

"Our family read this book together. Now we all have a point of reference when things get crazy. MOON is part of our family."

"It's like a tiny meditation, whenever I need it. And I need it a lot!"

"I'm less judgmental and my insight has deepened."

"I keep this book on my desk at work, sometimes on top of my computer. It's helped me and my clients in many situations."

"My test grades are higher."

I offer this information in hopes that your health and well being are refreshed and nurtured.

Books from Safe Goods Publishing
Order line: (888) NATURE-1

For a complete catalog of Safe Goods books call (888) NATURE-1 or look us up on the internet at: www.safegoodspub.com

The Brain Train	$4.95 US
Frances Meiser	$7.95 CAN
Low Carb and Beyond	$8.95 US
Nina Anderson & Dr Howard Peiper	$12.95 CAN
Overcoming Senior Moments	$7.95 US
Frances Meiser & Nina Anderson	$11.95 CAN
The Secrets of Staying Young	$ 9.95 US
Nina Anderson & Dr. Howard Peiper	$14.95 CAN
Stress and Weight Management using Rhodiola rosea &	$ 9.95 US
Rhododendron Caucasicum	$14.95 CAN
Dr. Zakir Ramazanov & Dr. Maria del Mar Bernal Suarez	
Natural Born Fatburners	$14.95 US
George Redmon, Ph.D., N.D	$19.95 CAN
Kiss Your Life Hello	$ 9.95 US
Dr. Howard Peiper	$14.95 CAN
2012 Airborne Prophesy	$16.95 US
A novel by Nina Anderson	$ 22.95 CAN
Spirit and Creator	$22.95 US
A photo documentary by Nova Hall	$34.50 CAN